Your Amazing Itty Bitty® How To Be A Woman Book

15 Easy Steps to Presenting Your Best Image!

!

Dr. Bunny Vreeland

Published by Itty Bitty® Publishing
A subsidiary of S & P Productions, Inc.
Copyright © 2016 **Dr. Bunny Vreeland**

Printed in the United States of America

Itty Bitty Publishing
311 Main Street, Suite D
El Segundo, CA 90245
(310) 640-8885

ISBN: 978-1-931191-12-8

Dedicated to all of my amazing women friends, mentors and teachers, who have touched & influenced my life in ways they may never know - specifically,

Marge Cavolt, the owner of Les Mannequinettes Modeling School, who taught me how to dress and walk without being self conscious,

Marje Thomas, an artist and interior designer, who taught me how to organize and put the pieces together,

Mary Michels, artist and college art teacher, who taught me line and color,

Norma Virgin, whose great Imagine and Color company, Beauty For All Seasons, paved the way for all of us image consultants.

Special acknowledgment to my incredible assistant of over 20 years, Sandi Buley. Sandi is my right hand, a dear friend and a perfect example of how to be a woman.

Stop by our Itty Bitty® website to find interesting blog entries regarding **How To Be A Woman.**

www.IttyBittyPublishing.com

Contact Dr. Bunny Vreeland at
Vreeland College of the Healing Arts
(805) 482-8111
E-mail: Bunny@BunnyVreeland.com

www.BunnyVreeland.org
www.VreelandCollege.org

Table of Contents

Introduction

In this Itty Bitty Book you will find all the components that come together to create YOUR total best look. By following the 15 easy-to-understand steps, you can discover that a great 'look' isn't created by one, singular image choice, but is instead made up of a series of choices.

When you're trying to decide what your next choice might be…

Two great questions to ask yourself are:

"Will this choice bring me closer to what I want?"

and

"Is this in alignment with the image I want to present?"

Step 1
Unleash Your Total Best Look

Style, Body Typing and Color are three components that come together to create your total best look. But, where can you find that total best look? Magazines and TV aren't any help. They are trying to sell stuff!

Start by discovering what you are attracted to. Or, think of someone whose body type is similar to yours and who has a style you admire.

1. Once you find someone whose style you admire, analyze it. Really look and break down what you like about it.
2. Check out fashion magazines that you are attracted to – InStyle, Vogue, Essence, Seventeen…..there are magazines for all types and all ages.
3. Cut out the pictures and create a collection. Compare them so you can see what it is that you like. What are the constants?

Guidelines

Because your total best look comes together with Style, Body Typing and Color, there are a few important guidelines to keep in mind:

- Your look should be compatible with your lifestyle.
- It's possible to be a combination of two different styles (as in elegant and glamorous).
- Find your best features and accent them.
- Color is key – to wardrobe, makeup & hair coordinating!
- Create your unique fashion statement by mastering these key components!

Step 2
Rock Your First Impression!

When I first became an Image Consultant, the theory was that it took three minutes to make a first impression. A few years later, that time zoomed to 60 seconds, and then, seven seconds. In today's fast-paced world, it takes just one-tenth of a second for us to judge someone and make a first impression of them. Make YOURS great!

1. A first impression is created when one initially encounters another person and forms a mental image of them.
2. Other people form impressions of you based on a wide range of characteristics: age, physical appearance, posture, and voice, are just a few of them.
3. The first impressions individuals give could greatly influence how they are treated and viewed in everyday life.

Tips To Making A Great First Impression:

- Take notice of your physical appearance – a good haircut, a nice outfit and coordinated makeup are essential.
- Be yourself – the trick is to be consistently you, at your best. The most effective people never change character from one situation to another.
- Make eye contact – whether you're talking to one person or 100, always look at them.
- Smile – use your gentle, comfortable smile, not forced.
- Listen before talking – really listen to what the other person is saying before giving your response or opinion.
- Focus your energy – It's important to have an air of certainty. Properly focused energy has a magnetic intensity that we all display when we sincerely believe something.
- Lighten up – it's easy to spot someone who takes themselves too seriously. Be comfortable with you.

Step 3
Identify Your Personal Style

Your personal style is what looks best on YOU.

1. Your personal style is determined by your body line, height and contours.
2. Your personal style makes the most of your features and assets.
3. Your personal style fits with your lifestyle.
4. Personal style is just that – it's personal. What works for one person may not work for another.

Personal Style Determiners

To help determine your personal style, ask yourself, what image you want to project? Who do you relate to? Are you:

- Dramatic/Bold – Attention-getting, commanding, exaggerated consummate style. Examples: Cher, Diana Ross, Christina Aguilera
- Arty/Creative – Unusual way of putting clothing items together, one-of-a-kind, individualized. Examples: Madonna, Lady Gaga, Whoopi Goldberg
- Classic/Timeless – Traditional, conservative, practical. Examples: Diane Sawyer, Barbara Bush
- Casual/Sporty – Natural, wholesome, easy, youthful. Examples: Christy Brinkley, Kathy Ireland
- Feminine/Romantic – Soft, sweet, fragile and delicate. Examples: Jane Seymour, Angelina Jolie
- Sexy/Seductive – Sensuous, revealing, body-emphasizing. Examples: Dolly Parton, Raquel Welch
- Elegant/Sophisticated – Refined, understated, ladylike. Examples: Helen Mirren, Grace Kelly

Step 4
What's Your Body Type?

Here are some tips to help you identify your personal body type. Which shape do you most identify with?

1. Rectangle – Straight up & down figure. Waist is no more than 8 inches smaller than hips & bust. This is the body type of most models in magazines.
2. Triangle – Shoulders & bust are smaller than hips. Larger below the waist than above the waist. This is the classic pear shape & most common female body type.
3. Hourglass – Hips & bust are similar measurements. Waist is at least 9 inches smaller than hips or bust. This is the classic "Marilyn Monroe" figure.
4. Oval – Hips are no larger than bust. Lowest part of the hip is smaller than the rest of the hip area. This body type usually has slim, shapely legs.

Accent – Don't Judge

Your body type is your body type it can be
flattered by the clothes you choose it can't be
eliminated. Think of it as the marble out of which
Michel Angelo carved his gorgeous statues – the
starting point.

- Start with a great foundation. A good
  fitting bra and undergarments are
  essential.
- Every woman has the potential to be
  perfectly satisfied with herself no matter
  what her size, height or age.
- Petite or Plus-Size, short or tall, you can
  learn to accent the best and camouflage
  the rest.
- Find your best feature and show it off.
- Each Body Type has its positives and
  challenges. No body is perfect.
- The mirror won't lie. Use it.

Step 5
The Best Colors For You!

Color and Image consulting took the world by storm in the 80's, 90's and early 2000's. Everyone was having their 'colors done' because it was a shortcut to looking your best, while saving money and time. Color is the key to putting your wardrobe together.

There are complete books written on color and how to wear it. Here are some quick & easy guidelines:

1. Your best colors to wear are determined by the undertone of your skin, eyes and hair. Warm or Cool.
2. Follow your eye and hair color to bring out your best coloring.
3. Colors are divided into 4 'seasons' – Winter, Summer (both Cool undertones) and Spring and Autumn (both Warm undertones).
4. Everyone can wear almost every color, but the undertone is different for each 'season'.
5. There are 4 universal colors that everyone can confidently wear – they are cream, turquoise, coral and periwinkle.

Determining Your Undertone & Season

Although there are exceptions to everything, here are some quick guidelines to determining your undertone & Season:

5. If you have naturally dark hair, dark eyes & dark skin, you are likely a Winter (there are more Winters in the world than any other season).
6. If you have naturally ash blonde or ash brown hair, blue/grey or green/grey eyes & rosy skin, you are likely a Summer.
7. If you have naturally golden blonde, golden brown, or sometimes bright red hair, vibrant blue or green eyes, and ivory or warm peach skin, you are likely a Spring.
8. If you have naturally golden brown, chestnut or golden red hair, hazel, warm brown or green eyes, warm peach, beige or warm ivory skin, you are likely an Autumn.

Step 6
Create Magic With Your Best Colors

The colors that work best with the various seasons are:

1. Winters are best in true, primary colors – red-reds, blue-blues, nothing muted. Winter's light colors are true & icy – as if chalk white has been added to the basic primary color.
2. Summers are best in dusty tones of primary colors. As if you've taken a powder puff to the Winter colors and softened it. Summer's "own" the pastel family.
3. Springs are best in warm, or golden-undertoned colors. Clear, Spring bouquet shades. Light & lively colors make up the Spring color palette. Dark & heavy colors overwhelm the delicate Spring coloring.
4. Autumns are best in rich, warm, muted shades. Springs and Autumns are cousins and some of their colors might overlap – especially yellows, oranges and browns. Earthy shades are the foundation of an Autumn's color palette.

Capsule Colors & Accessory Tones

Each season has a "capsule" of three basic colors.
These are the colors you build your wardrobe
around. When you know your basic colors you
could get dressed in the dark & step out looking
ready to go!

9. Winter's capsule: black and icy white,
   with true red or true blue, as a
   complimentary color. Jewelry tone:
   Silver. Footwear: Black
10. Summer's capsule: camel or rose-brown
    and off-white, with powder pink or baby
    blue as complimentary color. Jewelry
    tone: silver and gold (Summer is the only
    season that can wear both successfully).
    Footwear: Soft brown or camel.
11. Spring's capsule: Navy blue or soft
    brown and ivory, with coral or soft
    yellow as complimentary color. Jewelry
    tone: Gold. Footwear: Navy blue.
12. Autumn's capsule: Chocolate brown or
    Rust and oyster white, with peach or light
    turquoise as complimentary color.
    Jewelry tone: Gold. Footwear: Brown

Step 7
Get Dressed In Five Minutes

Sometimes, I have an early appointment or meeting and it is still dark when I get up. I don't want to wake my husband so I literally get dressed in the walk-in closet – in the dark - if I didn't assemble my clothes, the night before.

Here is how I do it:

1. Tops and bottoms – This is where mix and match is really essential. If clothes are color-coordinated, you will be able to grab & go!
2. Complimentary colors – these are found opposite each other on the color wheel, such as red/green, black/white, purple/yellow, orange/blue.
3. Color blocks – these are blocks of color which can make you appear shorter, taller, slimmer or heavier, depending on how you wear them.
4. Capsule – Taking minimum amount of clothing & using them to get the maximum amount of looks.

A Capsule Wardrobe Defined:

A capsule wardrobe is a term first used in the 70's by a boutique owner in London. The idea was that having a collection of a few classic wardrobe pieces – such as pants, skirts and jackets – could be interchanged with seasonal pieces to create many looks.

- A capsule wardrobe is made up of only interchangeable items.
- With a capsule wardrobe, you can create an outfit for any occasion without the need for excessive purchases.
- A capsule wardrobe generally contains two pairs of pants, one skirt or dress, a coat, a jacket, a sweater, two pairs of shoes and two handbags.
- For longevity, always choose classic cuts and high quality fabrics.
- A capsule wardrobe should ALWAYS be in your color palette.

Step 8
What's Your Lifestyle?

To be truly happy with your wardrobe, you must be aware of your lifestyle. If your wardrobe works with your lifestyle, it's smooth sailing ahead! Here are some things to consider:

1. What do you do for a living? Are you a stay-at-home mother? Are you an attorney? Are you a tennis instructor? It's easy to see how your wardrobe must be compatible with your lifestyle!
2. What kinds of clothes do you need for your daily life? A full-time professional, for example, needs a different wardrobe than someone who works part-time, or is retired.
3. How much of your time is spent in casual attire? Or professional or dressy attire?
4. What is your wardrobe budget? Depending on your budget, you can build your capsule wardrobe in as little as three months.
5. How much closet space do you have? A cluttered closet is not your friend!

What's Missing From Your Wardrobe?

Now that you're thinking about how your lifestyle affects your wardrobe, let's see what may be missing from your closet. Consider this:

13. How is the majority of your time spent? In a typical day, how is your time divided between professional time, home time, family time and recreation?
14. Look at your current wardrobe. Make a list of the amount of clothing you have for professional time, home time, family time and recreation.
15. Compare the time spent on a typical day with the amount of clothing you have for each category.
16. Make a list of what's missing. Do you have more professional clothes, but very little clothing for recreation? This is an easy way to create a shopping list of things you need to complete your wardrobe.

Step 9
Boost Your Attitude

Attitude is everything! It makes the difference between a good day/bad day and even a good life/bad life! Here are some tips to boost your attitude:

1. Move your body – even taking a walk in the morning can start your day off right!
2. Compliment at least one person everyday – see the beauty in someone else and make them smile. It's contagious!
3. Surround yourself with positive people!
4. Fake it 'til you make it! When you act enthusiastic, you will soon be enthusiastic!
5. Stress can take its toll, so give it the boot! I listen to my stress reduction CDs whenever I'm feeling stressed. You can listen to it, too - for free! http://bunnyvreeland.org/free-stress-reduction-session/

More Tips For Boosting Your Attitude

There are thousands of ways to boost your attitude. Try a few and see what works for you!

17. Sleep! Getting the proper amount of sleep leaves you feeling refreshed & ready to go.
18. Start your day with breakfast. It really is the most important meal of the day & even just a smoothie can get you moving.
19. Help someone in need. Giving of yourself not only helps the other person, but makes you feel good, too. A win/win!!
20. Listen to music that makes you happy. Whether it's classical or rock 'n roll, if it lifts your spirits, you're on the right track!

Step 10
Put Your Best Skin Forward!

We all strive for beautiful, glowing skin! Make yours the best it can be by using these quick tips:

1. First determine your skin type. Oily, Dry, Combination or Normal.
2. Find the products that work best for your skin type. If you're not sure, you can usually find samples to try at the major department stores, online or in specialty stores like Sephora. There are also trained consultants with companies like Mary Kay, Arbonne and Jafra, who will come to your home and instruct you on what types of products are best for you.
3. Wear a hat and sunscreen. Exposure to the sun is one of the most aging things you can do to your skin. There've been major improvements in sunscreen over the years – it's not the pore-clogging, greasy mess is used to be. You can even get sunscreen in powder form!

More Tips To Putting Your Best Skin Forward:

It's easy to create a simple skin care routine that works for you! Here are the steps to include in your daily routine:

- Cleanse
- Tone
- Moisturize
- Once a week use an exfoliator to slough off dead skin & uncover new, radiate skin underneath!

There's a product for every skin type, but the price of products can vary greatly. Keep in mind that you don't have to spend a fortune – moderately priced products are frequently wonderful! And remember – samples are a great way to determine what works for you, before investing in a full-size bottle.

Step 11
Make-up Tips And Tricks

Wearing makeup can take as little as five minutes and be very simple. Here are 4 easy steps to quickly enhance your natural features:

1. Eyebrows – Have them professionally shaped. Using brow pencil will help fill any gaps. Brows give balance to your face & frame your eyes.
2. Use mascara and eyeliner to define the shape of your eyes & make them stand out.
3. Applying blush to your cheeks gives your complexion a healthy glow and adds dimension to your cheekbones.
4. Lip color is the finishing touch that completes your look. Lip color defines the shape of your mouth and gives your lips definition.
5. A light application of foundation or face powder helps even out your skin tone.

More Make-up Tips And Tricks

You can apply your makeup any way you want. I usually start at the top and work my way down, so I don't forget anything. Consider your face as a palette and you are the artist.

- After you cleanse and moisturize, apply foundation.
- To determine your correct foundation color, apply a small amount to your jawline and blend downward. If the color seems to disappear, you've got the right color.
- Shape and fill in your eyebrows.
- Use eyeliner to define your eyes & bring out their beauty.
- Mascara makes your eyes look awake and alive. It is really a key to a pretty and polished look.
- Lip liner and lipstick add the finishing touch, defining your lips and adding color.

Step 12
Hairstyles For Your Face Shape!

How do you find the hairstyle that's best for your face shape? The basic rule is to never highlight your problem spot. Here's where to start:

1. **Oval faces** – Oval faces are usually compatible with most hairstyles, but they can appear long. Beware of adding too much height to the top of the head. If you have curly or thick hair, avoid blunt cuts which give the pyramid affect.
2. **Square faces** – texture, such as curls, helps to soften your strong, angular jaw. Have your hairstylist create long layers that go inward, rather than outward.
3. **Round face** – A haircut that hits below the chin, or longer, is ideal. Be sure to avoid wavy or short styles, as these will make the face appear rounder.
4. **Heart-shaped face** – Generally has a chin that comes to a point. Bring attention to your eyes and cheekbones with long side-swept bangs, a short pixy cut or long, choppy bob.

Ever Tried A Wig?

If you're unsure about your face shape or hair color, visit a wig boutique. Try on different wig colors and styles – short, long, curly, straight, blonde, brunette, red…. You'll be amazed at what might look great on you that you may not have considered before!

- Look for a wig expert – someone who can see things in you that you might not see in yourself.
- Keep an open mind. A particular style might look amazing on you, even though you're not ready to make the leap to that particular cut or color. It will still inspire you to see the other sides of yourself and the possibilities for future styles.
- Consider purchasing a wig you like & wearing it for a couple of weeks before you cut or color your hair in that style.
- Consider purchasing a wig just for the fun of it and for a change of pace! It's a great way to get ready faster and have a new look, too!

Step 13
Find Your 'Happy' And Share It

There are many versions of happy. There's 'quick happy' – as in "let's eat an ice cream cone", but that is not necessarily long-term happy. And there is a "long term happy."

When you strive to find your inner (long term) happiness, it begins to show outwardly – and it's contagious! It can be anything from yoga to bike riding to meditation to writing in a journal or volunteering.

Here are a few tips to spark your inspiration:

1. Do you feel best when helping others?
2. Is fresh air & exercise your idea of an ideal day?
3. Do you feel rejuvenated from quiet moments of inward reflection?
4. Do you find joy spending time with cats or dogs or horses?

Think about those moments where you really felt true joy, happiness & bliss – that is the place to start!

Ways To Find Your 'Happy'

Here are some more tips to 'find your happy':

- Many times happiness comes from finding something bigger than yourself. It takes the spotlight off of your own issues, and puts the focus on helping other people.
- Exercise boosts your endorphins – your body's natural happiness chemical.
- Surround yourself with positive people. Like I mentioned before, happiness is contagious!
- Eliminate as much negativity in your life as possible.
- Smile! When you smile at other people, they smile back & it creates more 'happy' for everyone!

Step 14
Putting The Pieces Together

When I was an Image Consultant, I learned
2 pieces of information that impacted me the
most and have stuck with me over the years:

1. Most of us wear between 20-25% of our
   wardrobe. Think about that. Stand in
   front of your closet. Does that ring true
   for you and your wardrobe?
2. We waste over $65,000.00 in makeup
   and wardrobe mistakes, in our lifetime,
   by buying items that don't flatter our
   body and/or don't go with anything else
   in our closet. 50% off a gorgeous piece of
   clothing is not a 'deal' unless you can use
   it.

Anyone with a credit card can walk into a store
an emerge looking like a Fashionista. But very
few people – credit cards or not – can be
considered a woman of genuine style.
When you know how to put the pieces – color,
body type, makeup, hairstyle, personal style and
lifestyle – together, you will find that your
wardrobe works FOR you and saves you
time, money and frustration.

Things To Keep In Mind When Shopping:

- Your colors! Is that item in your color palette?
- Your lifestyle! Can you wear that item often?
- Your body type! Is that item flattering to your figure?

Things To Keep In Mind When Clearing Out Your Closet:

- Is that item out of style? Is it classic enough to come back into style?
- Is it repairable, or beyond repair?
- Make 3 piles – Keep, Discard, Repair.
- When was the last time you wore that? If it's been over a year, you might consider donating it to a friend or charity.

Step 15
Looking Ahead

If you have been alive for any amount of time or traveled to any area of the world, you know that fashion is in a constant state of flux. The only thing constant is change. So, rather than trying to guess what might be in our fashion future, let's concentrate on some basics. These basics will always be important, whether you embrace Shabby Chic or Ultra Trendy.

1. Dental care – see your dentist at least every 6 months. Beautiful smiles are always in fashion.
2. Hygiene – even the most beautiful outfit won't cover up poor hygiene.
3. Regular checkups with a doctor – feeling good and looking good go hand in hand.
4. Foundation garments – the foundation is everything! Start with great undergarments and build from there.
5. Grooming – regular hair and nail appointments should be part of your regime.

The Foundation Is Everything

What is under your clothing sets the stage for a completed look. Here are some key tips to remember:

- Consider being professionally fitted to find your correct bra size. Your bra size will change over the years due to childbirth, weight and lifestyle changes.
- Consider shapewear to smooth your silhouette. There are some great types of shapewear these days that are very comfortable, unlike the old-fashioned girdle.
- Be sure to wear light colored foundations when wearing light colored clothing, so that the foundations don't show through.

You've finished. Before you go...

<u>Tweet/share that you finished this book.</u>

Please star rate this book.

Reviews are solid gold to writers. Please take a few minutes to give us some itty bitty feedback.

ABOUT THE AUTHOR

Dr. Bunny Vreeland is a former professional model, an award winning Color and Image Consultant and, for the past 20+ years, a Board Certified, Clinical Hypnotherapist.

Dr. Bunny has been a featured guest on many TV and radio shows, and a popular keynote speaker at numerous venues. Her articles on image, stress, self-esteem and hypnotherapy have appeared in many publications. She had a successful two year run as the host of "The Dr. Bunny Show... Here's the Thing" on KKZZ AM 1400 in Ventura, CA.

She founded the Vreeland College of the Healing Arts in Camarillo, CA, and continues her private Clinical Hypnotherapy practice at her peaceful office, located in the college.

Dr. Bunny was a 16-year old high school drop-out who went back to school and received her Ph.D. at the age of 60. Consequently, she is especially interested in helping teens stay in school.

You can listen to The Ask Dr. Bunny Show on www.MercuryBroadcasting.net, where her focus is on health, wellness and positive living.

Vreeland College of the Healing Arts
(805) 482-8111

E-mail: Bunny@BunnyVreeland.com
www.BunnyVreeland.org
www.VreelandCollege.org

If you enjoyed this Itty Bitty® Book you might also like…

- **Your Amazing Itty Bitty® Weight Loss Book** – Suzy Prudden and Joan Meijer-Hirschland
- **Your Amazing Itty Bitty® Cancer Book** – Jacqueline Kreple
- **Your Amazing Itty Bitty® Self-Esteem Book** – Jade Elizabeth

Or many other Itty Bitty® Books available on line.

Where Do You Go To Find Out How YOU Can Look And Feel Your Best?

Have You Noticed That Some Women Intuitively Know How To Look Marvelous? Want To Learn the Secret?

What happened to all the guidelines? Ever since casual Friday became 'the norm', presenting yourself in a polished and professional way seems to have fallen to the wayside.

As a former model, one of the top Image Consultants in the nation, and a Board Certified Clinical Hypnotherapist, Dr. Bunny Vreeland brings her expertise – and life experience – together to give you 15 easy-to-follow steps to save time, money & frustration, while creating your best YOU!

You will learn:

- Your body type, and how to dress for it!
- The best hairstyles for your face shape!
- How to dress effortlessly & look polished in 5-minutes!

If you want to present yourself in the best possible way for all occasions, pick up a copy of this fun and informative book today, and experience how easy it can be to look your best!